DEALING WITH MONKEY POX

All You Need to Know about its Prevention and Management

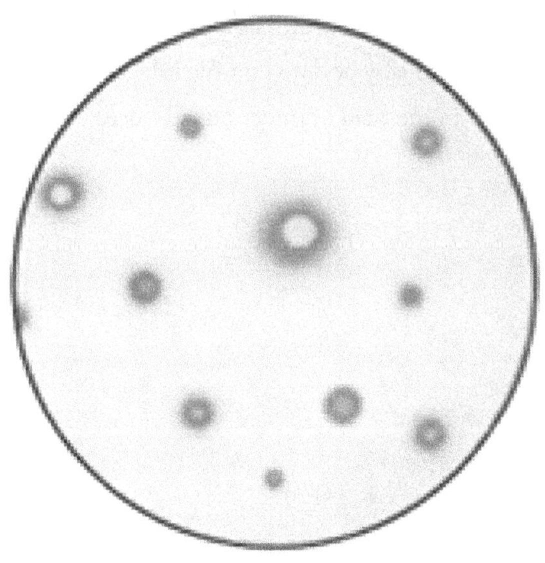

Philip Maximus

Copyright © 2023 Philip Maximus

All Rights Reserved

Table of Contents

Chapter 1: Introduction to Monkeypox

What is Monkeypox?

Monkeypox is a relatively uncommon and potentially life-threatening viral infection caused by a germ known as an orthopoxvirus. Its discovery dates back to 1958 when outbreaks were observed in laboratory monkeys, leading to the nomenclature "Monkeypox." This zoonotic illness has the capacity to cross over from animals to humans, manifesting in a range of symptoms from mild to severe. This section will delve into the particulars of Monkeypox, its origin, and its implications for human health.

The primary mode of transmission for Monkeypox to humans is through contact with infected animals, and while it is considered rare, it can give rise to epidemics in specific regions. The virus is most commonly found in Central and West Africa, with sporadic cases documented in other global locales. The primary reservoir hosts for the virus are believed to be rodents, particularly squirrels and monkeys, and human transmission can occur through direct contact with these animals or their bodily fluids.

Classified under the Orthopoxvirus genus, Monkeypox shares genetic similarities with well-known members such as Smallpox and Vaccinia virus. Despite the successful global eradication of Smallpox through vaccination, Monkeypox has proven to be a more formidable adversary.

Symptoms of Monkeypox in humans exhibit variability, ranging from mild illness to more severe complications. Common symptoms include fever, headache, muscular pains, backache, swollen lymph nodes, chills, and fatigue. A distinctive feature of Monkeypox is the development of a rash, typically starting on the face and spreading to other parts of the body. The rash progresses through stages, including the formation of fluid-filled pustules, often accompanied by intense itching.

While Monkeypox bears similarities to Smallpox, it generally presents with lower severity, boasting a mortality rate of less than 10%, in contrast to Smallpox's mortality rate of over 30%. Nonetheless, severe cases can arise, particularly in individuals with compromised immune systems. Early detection and diagnosis are imperative for providing timely medical intervention and curtailing further transmission.

Preventive measures for Monkeypox encompass several strategies. Currently, there exists no specific antiviral medication tailored for Monkeypox; however, supportive care can aid in symptom management. Formerly, Smallpox immunization was considered protective against Monkeypox, but the waning effectiveness of Smallpox vaccination, due to phased-down programs, has diminished this immunity. Ongoing research is focused on the development of a dedicated Monkeypox vaccine, though it is not yet accessible to the general public.

This information holds paramount importance for healthcare professionals, public health authorities, and the wider public, ensuring the swift identification and treatment of Monkeypox, thereby mitigating the impact of this intriguing yet formidable virus.

Monkeypox History

Let's look back at the story of Monkeypox, a mysterious virus with a history full of surprises and exploration. The tale of Monkeypox unfolds like a detective story, with each chapter revealing more about this puzzling virus and its complex relationship with humans.

The quest to uncover the origins of Monkeypox started in 1958, in an unexpected place: the United States. The story took place at a Missouri research center where scientists faced a series of mysterious outbreaks. These outbreaks didn't affect people but a group of caged monkeys from Africa. The symptoms shown by the monkeys, like skin lesions and pustules, were unique and unfamiliar to the scientific community.

In response, scientists launched an investigation to understand this new disease. They faced a pressing question: What caused these unusual diseases in the monkeys? This marked the beginning of Monkeypox.

The term "Monkeypox" was coined to name this peculiar illness discovered in monkeys. However, what was found in monkeys had a significant impact on our understanding of diseases that can pass from animals to humans.

In 1970, a groundbreaking discovery changed the Monkeypox story. The Democratic Republic of the Congo reported the first documented case of Monkeypox in humans. This was a crucial moment, revealing the virus's ability to jump from its natural hosts, like rodents and monkeys, to people. This aspect of the virus added to its intrigue and concern.

The virus causing Monkeypox belongs to the Orthopoxvirus group, which includes well-known viruses like Smallpox and Vaccinia. Smallpox had a major impact on human history, causing widespread death and suffering until it was eradicated through vaccination efforts. Scientists were intrigued by the genetic similarities between Monkeypox and Smallpox, wanting to understand their connection and how Monkeypox differs in terms of severity and transmission.

Monkeypox's history is marked by scientific breakthroughs and challenges. Researchers have worked hard to unravel the virus's mysteries, from its origins in African animals to its spread to human populations. The complexities of the Monkeypox story underscore the importance of ongoing research and vigilance in monitoring potential outbreaks.

As we explore the chapters of Monkeypox history, we realize that the story is far from over. It's a tale of discovery, persistence, and the ongoing effort to comprehend a virus that continues to present challenges and uncertainty in the fields of medicine and public health. Understanding the historical background of Monkeypox is crucial for healthcare professionals, academics, and the general public as we strive to combat and manage this viral illness.

Monkeypox vs. Smallpox

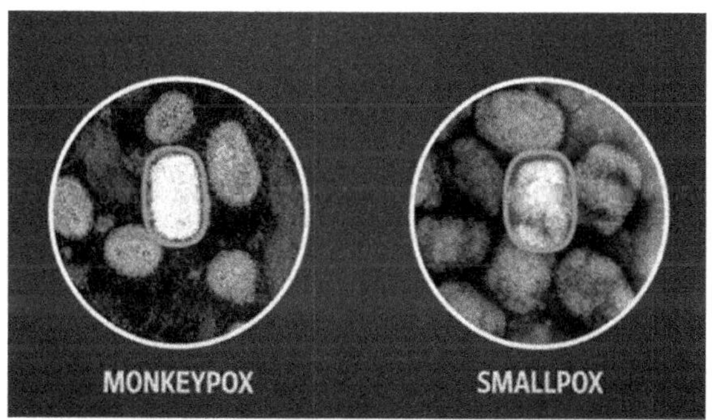

Understanding the differences between similar viruses in the context of infectious diseases is like solving a challenging puzzle. One interesting comparison is between smallpox and monkeypox. These two viruses share genetic similarities, have historical importance, and can infect humans. However, they also have significant differences that impact how they affect public health. Let's explore the details and distinctions between smallpox and monkeypox in this section.

Before we dive into the comparison, let's briefly look at the history of these viruses. The World Health Organization led a global vaccination effort that successfully eradicated smallpox in 1980, putting an end to a disease that had affected people for a long time. This achievement highlighted the effectiveness of vaccinations and public health efforts. In contrast, monkeypox was mostly unknown and only known to harm animals until human cases started appearing in the latter part of the 20th century.

One key difference between the two diseases is their fatality rates. Smallpox had a well-known high mortality rate, ranging from 20% to 30% for common cases and even higher for severe ones. In contrast, monkeypox generally has a lower death rate, estimated to be less than 10%. This distinction emphasizes that, while still concerning, monkeypox usually results in fewer fatalities compared to its more infamous relative, smallpox.

These diseases also differ in how they manifest clinically. Smallpox symptoms typically followed a predictable pattern, with survivors often left with severe scarring. Symptoms included a high fever, a distinctive rash, and the development of pustules. Monkeypox symptoms, on the other hand, are more varied. The pox-like rash, a characteristic sign of the disease, can be challenging to diagnose early on because the initial symptoms may resemble those of common illnesses like the flu.

The geographical distribution of the viruses is another point of difference. Smallpox posed a global threat, affecting people on nearly every continent. It was eventually eradicated through a worldwide immunization campaign. In contrast, monkeypox cases are sporadically reported outside of Central and West Africa, where the disease is primarily found. Understanding this spatial divide is crucial for focusing preventative and surveillance efforts in the right areas.

Vaccination has played a crucial role in the history of both viruses. The smallpox vaccine provided protection against both smallpox and, to some extent, monkeypox, contributing to the eradication of smallpox. However, since regular smallpox vaccination stopped, immunity has decreased, leaving the population more vulnerable to monkeypox. Efforts are underway to develop a specific vaccine for monkeypox to provide better defense against this new threat.

Monkeypox has a lower death rate than other comparable illnesses such as smallpox. The majority of instances are mild and self-limiting, and deaths are uncommon.

Chapter 2: Understanding Monkey Pox Transmission and Symptoms

Monkeypox is a rare but serious viral illness that is closely related to smallpox. It's a zoonotic disease, meaning it can be passed from animals to people. The main animals carrying the Monkeypox virus are wild animals, especially rodents, and these animals are believed to keep the virus in their populations in Africa.

After the virus passes from animals to people, it can then spread from person to person. Monkeypox is mainly transmitted through:

a) Direct Contact with Infected Animals:
Getting Monkeypox can happen by touching
infected animals, like handling their bodies or
being bitten or scratched. This type of
transmission is more common in places where
hunting and eating wild animals are part of the
local culture.

b) Person-to-Person Transmission: This
type of transmission occurs when someone
with Monkeypox is in close contact with others.
The virus can spread through respiratory
droplets when an infected person coughs,
sneezes, or talks. Direct contact with an
infected person's skin sores or body fluids can
also lead to transmission.

c) Object Transmission: Monkeypox can
also spread indirectly through objects. Objects
or surfaces, like clothes, bedding, or items used
by an infected person, can carry the virus.
Touching these contaminated items and then

touching your face, eyes, nose, or mouth could make you sick.

d) Hospital Transmission: There's a risk of Monkeypox spreading in healthcare settings to healthcare workers and other patients. To prevent this, it's crucial to follow strict infection control measures, like isolating sick people and using protective gear.

e) Animal Contact Transmission: This type of transmission occurs when people come into contact with infected animals. It's a concern for those living near natural areas or engaging in activities that involve contact with animals carrying the virus.

Understanding these ways of transmission is vital for implementing effective preventive measures. Taking steps like avoiding contact with wild animals and following safety measures in medical settings can help reduce the risk of Monkeypox transmission. If there's a suspected outbreak, quickly isolating affected individuals and tracing their contacts can help limit the spread of the virus.

Common Symptoms

Now that we've talked about how Monkeypox spreads, let's look at the usual signs of this sickness. Knowing these signs is important for getting the right help on time.

Monkeypox usually takes 5 to 21 days to show symptoms after you catch the virus. The symptoms can be mild or severe, and they might seem like those of other sicknesses, making it hard to know without proper testing. Monkeypox shows these signs:

Fever: Monkeypox often starts with a high fever, reaching 101°F (38.3°C) or more. This fever is one of the first signs and can last for several days.

Headache: People with Monkeypox often get strong headaches, which can be really bad. The headache might feel different for each person.

Muscle Aches: Monkeypox brings muscle aches and overall body discomfort, similar to the flu.

Chills and Sweating: Many Monkeypox patients feel chills and sweat a lot. Going from chills to sweating can make things more uncomfortable.

Fatigue: Feeling tired and weak is common with Monkeypox. Patients often feel exhausted and may find it hard to do their daily tasks.

Swollen Lymph Nodes: Monkeypox often causes swollen lymph nodes in the neck, groin, and armpit areas.

Skin Lesions: Monkeypox shows tiny bumps on the skin that fill with fluid and turn into pustules. These lesions appear on the face, trunk, and limbs, often forming crusts and scabs.

Rash: Along with skin lesions, a rash may appear which can be painful. For doctors, the rash is an important sign for diagnosis.

Remember, Monkeypox affects people differently. In some cases, it goes away on its own without treatment. But in severe cases, problems like pneumonia, eye infections, and rarely, death, can occur.

Monkeypox symptoms can be mistaken for other infections like chickenpox or measles. That's why it's crucial to seek medical help if you have these symptoms, especially if you've been close to someone with Monkeypox or have been to places where it's known.

Doctors usually confirm Monkeypox through lab tests on blood, skin, or other fluids. Finding it early and treating it is important to manage symptoms, prevent issues, and reduce the risk of spreading it more.

Monkeypox and Those at Risk

Now, let's focus on understanding which groups of people are more likely to get monkeypox. This helps us pay extra attention to those who need protection the most. Identifying these vulnerable groups is important for creating personalized plans to prevent and deal with the virus.

People Close to Infected Animals: If you live in or near places where monkeypox is common in wildlife, you might be at a higher risk. This includes communities that hunt, capture, or deal with wild animals because they might have direct contact with sick animals or their fluids.

Healthcare Workers: Those who take care of patients with monkeypox are more likely to come into contact with the virus. Healthcare workers may touch patients' fluids, so it's crucial to have strict infection control rules, like using protective gear, in healthcare places.

Close Contacts with Infected People: If you're close to someone with monkeypox, like friends, family, or caretakers, you could be at risk. The virus can spread through direct contact with skin sores, body fluids, and even through the air when someone breathes. Isolating affected people quickly can reduce the risk to close contacts.

Visitors to Risky Areas: Travelers going to places where monkeypox is common or outbreaks are happening have a higher risk. Important precautions for travelers include avoiding contact with wild animals, keeping good hygiene, and knowing the symptoms.

People with Weak Immune Systems: Those getting cancer treatment, organ transplants, HIV/AIDS patients, and others with weakened immune systems are more likely to get seriously sick from monkeypox. Their bodies may struggle to fight the infection because their immune systems are not as strong.

Children: While kids might not be more likely to get monkeypox, if they do, they could have a more serious infection. Parents and caregivers should be careful to spot symptoms in children and get medical help quickly.

Non-Immune Populations: In places where monkeypox isn't common and people haven't been exposed to it before, there might be no immunity. If the virus gets introduced in these areas, it could lead to more serious outbreaks.

Understanding these at-risk groups is crucial to stop monkeypox from spreading. Customized preventive actions can help reduce the risks. This includes vaccination campaigns for healthcare workers, educating communities in risky areas about public health, and making sure travelers are aware.

Here are some ways to prevent monkeypox for at-risk groups:

- Avoid contact with wild animals in risky areas, especially rats.
- Keep good hygiene by using hand sanitizers and washing hands regularly.
- Encourage healthcare workers to wear protective gear.
- Promote vaccination in areas where monkeypox is common.
- Isolate and quarantine suspected cases quickly to stop the infection from spreading.

By identifying and addressing the populations more likely to get monkeypox, we can try to

reduce the impact of this virus and protect the
health of those who are most vulnerable.

Chapter 3: Prevention and Vaccination

Vaccination plays a big role in the fight against contagious sicknesses like monkeypox, keeping people and communities safe. Vaccination, named after the Latin word "vacca" meaning cow (thanks to Edward Jenner's work with cowpox), is a preventive treatment that has saved many lives over time.

Understanding Vaccination:

Vaccination is when a weakened or inactive form of a germ (like the Monkeypox virus) is put into the body. This exposure helps the immune system make antibodies and memory cells without causing sickness. So, if a vaccinated person encounters the real virus, their immune system is ready to fight it off, either preventing it or making the sickness less severe.

Types of Vaccines:

There are different vaccines used against monkeypox. Here are a few examples:

Live Attenuated Vaccines: These have a weakened but still alive form of the Monkeypox virus. For instance, the smallpox vaccination can offer some protection against monkeypox. However, they can be risky for people with weakened immune systems.

Inactivated or Killed Vaccines: These use a non-live, inactive form of the virus. They are usually less risky, but might need booster doses to keep immunity.

Protein Subunit Vaccines: Instead of the whole virus, these vaccines contain pure parts of the virus, like proteins. They are often safer but may require adjuvants (things that boost the body's immune response).

Viral Vector Vaccines: These vaccines use a harmless virus to carry genetic material from the Monkeypox virus into the body, prompting an immune response. This method has shown promise in recent vaccine development.

Vaccination Programs: Governments and healthcare groups often run vaccination programs to control monkeypox outbreaks and prevent future cases. These programs focus on vulnerable groups like healthcare workers, people in affected areas, and those in close contact with confirmed cases. They often use a ring vaccination approach, vaccinating not only the sick person but also those nearby.

Vaccination Challenges: Even though vaccination is crucial for preventing monkeypox, there are challenges to overcome. Some people can't get vaccinated due to allergies or health issues. Also, fears and false information about vaccines can hinder vaccination efforts. Dealing with these issues through public education is important.

To sum up, vaccination measures are essential to prevent Monkeypox. Different vaccines are used, and vaccination programs aim to protect vulnerable groups. Overcoming challenges like contraindications and vaccine hesitancy is vital for these strategies to work effectively.

Staying Safe from Monkeypox

Staying safe from Monkeypox is really important to prevent getting sick and spreading the virus to others. While getting vaccinated is a good first step, there are also simple things you can do every day to stay safe and protect yourself and those around you.

Washing Hands and Keeping Things Clean: One of the best ways to stop Monkeypox from spreading is by washing your hands regularly with soap and water for at least 20 seconds. If you can't find soap and water, using hand sanitizers with at least 60% alcohol can also help. Don't forget to clean things you touch a lot, like doorknobs, phones, and keyboards. And remember; try not to touch your face, especially your eyes, nose, and mouth.

Wearing Face Masks and Covering Up: Wearing a face mask is a good idea when you're close to people, like in crowded places or if you're taking care of someone with Monkeypox. Masks help keep virus droplets from spreading. Also, cover your mouth and nose with a tissue or your elbow when you cough or sneeze, and throw used tissues in the trash. Wash your hands right after.

Keeping Your Distance: It's smart to stay away from people who might have Monkeypox symptoms or are confirmed cases. Avoid things like hugs, handshakes, or standing too close to someone who might be sick. By keeping a safe distance, you lower the chance of catching the virus directly.

Keeping Things Clean Around You: Cleaning and disinfecting things you touch a lot, like doorknobs and shared gadgets can help a lot. Use cleaning products that work against viruses like Monkeypox and follow the instructions on the label.

Taking Care of Yourself: If you think you might have been near someone with Monkeypox or if you're feeling sick with symptoms like fever, rash, or swollen lymph nodes, it's important to stay away from others. Get medical help and tests to see if you have the virus. Health officials might also ask you to stay away from others for a while to stop the virus from spreading.

Using Protective Gear: If you work in healthcare or have to be close to someone with Monkeypox, it's important to wear the right protective gear, like gloves, gowns, masks, and face shields. This gear helps keep you safe from getting the virus while taking care of someone who's sick.

Doing these things every day is a smart way to protect yourself and your community from Monkeypox. Remember, your actions make a difference in keeping everyone safe from contagious illnesses. It's a team effort, and every person plays a part in staying healthy.

Staying Safe from Monkeypox

Quarantine and isolation are important steps in keeping infectious diseases like monkeypox under control. They help prevent the virus from spreading and protect people from getting sick. These actions are meant to stop the illness from spreading and keep everyone healthy.

Understanding Quarantine and Isolation: In dealing with diseases like monkeypox, quarantine and isolation are two different but related ideas, each with a specific purpose.

Quarantine: Quarantine is a way to keep an eye on people who have been near someone with a contagious disease but haven't shown any symptoms yet. The goal is to watch them closely and limit their movement in case they start showing signs of the virus. This usually happens during the incubation period, which is the time between being exposed to the virus and getting sick. For monkeypox, this period can be anywhere from 5 to 21 days.

Isolation: Isolation is about separating people who are already sick and showing symptoms from those who are not sick. This helps stop the virus from spreading to others. Isolation continues until the person is no longer contagious and doesn't pose a risk to others.

When and Why Quarantine and Isolation Are Needed:

Quarantine and isolation are crucial for dealing with monkeypox for several reasons:

Containment: By isolating people who have been exposed and those who are confirmed to have the virus, the spread of the virus can be stopped, preventing new cases.

Protection: Isolation protects those who are sick from getting others sick. It ensures they get the right medical care and prevents the illness from spreading to their friends, family, and the community.

Observation: Quarantine allows close observation of people who have been near confirmed cases. This helps identify symptoms early, and they can get medical help quickly if needed.

Self-Isolation and Home Quarantine

These are important steps to take when dealing with monkeypox. Here's how to do them effectively:

Confirmed Cases: If you've been diagnosed with monkeypox, it's crucial to isolate yourself. If possible, use a separate bathroom and stay in a well-ventilated room away from other family members. If you have to be around others, wear a mask and follow good respiratory hygiene. As advised by your healthcare expert, avoid close contact with pets.

Home Quarantine for Exposed Individuals: If you've been in close contact with a confirmed case of monkeypox, you might need to stay at home in quarantine. Stay away from people, don't share personal items, and keep an eye on your health. Let medical authorities know if you develop any symptoms.

Community and Medical Facility Isolation: In more serious cases, people with severe symptoms of monkeypox may need to be isolated in medical facilities. This is especially important for those with serious symptoms or complications. Isolation rooms are set up to provide proper care and prevent the illness from spreading.

Support and Mental Health: Being in isolation or under quarantine can be tough emotionally. It's important to provide access to mental health resources and emotional support. Stay digitally connected with loved

ones and engage in activities that reduce stress
and anxiety.

Ongoing monkeypox research adds to a better knowledge of the virus, which aids in the development of better therapies and prevention measures. Increased awareness aids in early diagnosis and case

Chapter 4: Diagnosing Monkey Pox

Quick and accurate diagnosis is crucial for effective management and control. We'll break down the diagnostic process into three parts: clinical assessment, laboratory testing, and differential diagnosis.

Clinical Assessment

When you or someone you know shows symptoms that might be Monkeypox, the first step in figuring out the illness is a complete clinical evaluation. A healthcare professional, usually a doctor, will gather a lot of information about the patient's medical history and current symptoms during this process.

The healthcare professional might ask about recent travel, exposure to possible sources of infection, and any existing health issues. Pay close attention to these questions and be as honest as possible; your answers play a big role in the diagnostic process.

Fever, headache, muscle pains, and pox-like skin lesions are some key signs of Monkeypox that may be noticed during this evaluation. The healthcare professional will also ask about when these symptoms started and how they have progressed.

Next comes the physical examination. The doctor will carefully check the patient, focusing on any skin lesions, lymph nodes, and mucous membranes. Monkeypox often shows up as pox-like lesions that go through stages, similar to chickenpox. Monkeypox is identified by the presence of deep-seated, fluid-filled vesicles, which can help distinguish it from other infections.

As the patient, be ready to explain your symptoms, when they started, and any possible exposure to viral sources. This information is crucial if you've been in contact with animals, especially rodents like squirrels or monkeys, or people with Monkeypox.

The clinical examination is the first step in the diagnostic process and is crucial for spotting suspected Monkeypox cases. Keep in mind that Monkeypox is rare, and misdiagnoses happen because it looks like other viral diseases. So, your active participation in this process is crucial.

Be open about your recent activities, trips, and any contact with animals during the clinical examination. Also, make sure to provide any relevant medical documents or information about your health history. This teamwork between you and your healthcare provider sets the stage for the next steps in diagnosing Monkeypox.

Monkeypox Testing

After the initial checkup, testing in a lab is important to figure out if someone has Monkeypox. This step involves specific tests to confirm the presence of the Monkeypox virus in the patient's body. Lab testing is crucial for Monkeypox diagnosis because it provides strong evidence and helps distinguish the virus from other similar illnesses.

One of the main lab tests used for Monkeypox is the polymerase chain reaction (PCR) assay. PCR is a science method that magnifies and identifies the Monkeypox virus's genetic material, especially its DNA. This method allows the virus to be found early in blood, serum, or skin samples. PCR tests are sensitive and accurate, making them an important tool for confirming Monkeypox.

During lab testing, different samples like blood, swabs from skin sores, or scabs from pox-like sores may be taken. These samples are then sent to a specialized lab for examination. The results of the PCR test usually come back in a few days and can give a clear diagnosis.

While lab testing is crucial for confirming Monkeypox, it's important to know that PCR tests might not be available in every healthcare place. In such cases, patients might be sent to labs with the right equipment and expertise to do these tests correctly.

The lab testing process might seem complex, but it's important for ruling out other illnesses and getting a definite diagnosis. Once Monkeypox is confirmed through lab testing, the right treatment and isolation steps can be taken quickly.

If you find out you have Monkeypox, it's normal to be worried and have questions.

Keeping in touch with your healthcare provider is crucial in this situation. They will guide you through the process and explain the next steps, which might include staying in the hospital, isolation, and taking antiviral drugs to treat the illness.

Following the suggested treatment plan and working with healthcare experts is important if you're diagnosed with Monkeypox. This helps prevent the virus from spreading to others. Knowing that Monkeypox is a rare illness that needs special treatment will keep you informed and ready.

Identifying Monkeypox: Understanding Different Signs

Differential diagnosis is a crucial step in figuring out if someone has Monkeypox. During this stage, healthcare professionals use their knowledge to tell Monkeypox apart from other illnesses that share similar signs. Since Monkeypox has features similar to various viral illnesses, getting this step right is important for a proper diagnosis.

When patients show symptoms like fever, headache, muscle pains, and distinct pox-like skin sores, healthcare practitioners have to consider various possible reasons. Examples include chickenpox, smallpox, shingles, and other viral illnesses. The challenge is telling them apart because they might look the same.

One distinguishing factor in the diagnosis is the patient's history of exposure to potential sources of the virus. If the patient recently visited or lives where Monkeypox cases are known or had contact with animals like rats or monkeys, this information is crucial.

Doctors closely watch how the skin sores progress. Monkeypox sores go through stages, including papules, vesicles, pustules, and scabs. These sores look different, which can help tell Monkeypox apart from similar illnesses.

As mentioned earlier, lab testing is vital in the differential diagnosis. While symptoms may be similar to other illnesses, testing for Monkeypox viral DNA gives a definite diagnosis.

Patients might be asked to share detailed information about recent activities and possible exposures. This, combined with clinical evaluation and lab test results, helps create an informed diagnosis.

It's important to know that misdiagnosis can happen, especially in places where healthcare professionals may not be familiar with Monkeypox due to its rarity. Misdiagnoses could lead to delays in proper treatment and isolation, making it crucial to collaborate with your healthcare provider during the diagnostic process.

If Monkeypox is confirmed, treatment and containment measures can start immediately. This might include isolation to prevent the virus from spreading, antiviral drugs to treat the illness, and supportive care to ease symptoms.

Smallpox vaccination has demonstrated modest protection against monkeypox. This might perhaps lessen the severity of the sickness or avert it entirely.

Chapter 5: Treating Monkey Pox

Whether you're a healthcare professional or someone looking for information on handling Monkeypox, this chapter will provide essential insights into treatment options. The three main parts of Monkeypox therapy are Supportive Care, Antiviral Medications, and Managing Complications.

Supportive Care

Supportive care is a crucial aspect of Monkeypox treatment. It plays a vital role in easing symptoms, promoting healing, and reducing the risk of complications. Understanding the basics of supportive care is important for both patients and caregivers.

Supportive care involves addressing the symptoms and consequences of Monkeypox while the body's immune system fights the infection. Here are some key components of supportive care:

Isolation and Quarantine: Isolating the sick person is essential to prevent the spread of Monkeypox. Those who have had direct contact with the sick person should also be quarantined to monitor for symptoms.

Hydration: Staying hydrated is crucial, especially when fever and other symptoms lead to fluid loss. Drinking water, oral rehydration treatments, and intravenous fluids may be necessary.

Pain Management: Monkeypox often causes significant pain, such as muscle aches, joint discomfort, and headaches. Over-the-counter pain medicines like acetaminophen or ibuprofen can help, but proper doses should be determined by a healthcare professional.

Fever Control: Monkeypox is marked by high fever. Fever-reducing drugs, under medical supervision, can help lower body temperature.

Skin Care: Monkeypox results in distinctive skin sores that can be uncomfortable. Cleaning the skin and using soothing lotions or ointments may help. Avoid touching the sores to prevent further infections.

Nutritional Support: A healthy diet rich in vitamins and minerals aids in recovery. Liquid supplements may be recommended if eating is challenging due to a sore throat or mouth ulcers.

Psychological Support: Dealing with Monkeypox can be emotionally challenging. Emotional support and therapy can assist patients and their families in coping with the stress and worry.

As Monkeypox severity varies, personalized supportive treatment regimens from healthcare specialists are crucial. Close monitoring is necessary to identify and address issues promptly.

Supportive care forms the foundation of Monkeypox management, and a compassionate approach is essential for patient well-being. Whether you're a healthcare practitioner or caregiver, your support and compassion can make a significant impact on a patient's recovery journey.

Antiviral Medications

An essential part of Monkeypox treatment involves the use of antiviral drugs. These medications are designed to directly combat the Monkeypox virus, preventing it from reproducing within the body. This section will discuss the role of antiviral drugs and how they contribute to the treatment process.

Understanding Antiviral Medications:

Antiviral medicines are specialized pharmaceuticals crafted to combat viral infections. They function by disrupting the virus's ability to replicate and spread, allowing the body's immune system to more effectively combat the infection. In the case of Monkeypox, antiviral drugs play a crucial role in mitigating the severity and duration of the illness.

When Are Antiviral Medications Used?

The use of antiviral drugs is typically reserved for severe cases or individuals at a higher risk of complications from Monkeypox. Decisions regarding the administration of these drugs are made based on an individual's medical history and the progression of the condition.

Common Antiviral Medications:

While there is a variety of antiviral drugs available, the specific medication used to treat Monkeypox may vary. Cidofovir, a well-known antiviral medicine, has demonstrated promise in reducing the severity of Monkeypox. Another potential option is Brincidofovir, a newer antiviral medication showing effectiveness against Monkeypox.

Administration and Monitoring:

Antiviral drugs are typically administered intravenously, meaning they are injected directly into the bloodstream. This method allows for the rapid and targeted distribution of the antiviral medication throughout the body. Healthcare providers determine the dosage and duration of therapy based on the individual's condition.

While antiviral drugs can be beneficial in combating the Monkeypox virus, they also come with potential serious side effects that require careful monitoring. Close communication between the patient and healthcare practitioner is crucial to adjust the treatment as needed and address any adverse effects.

Potential Benefits and Limitations:

Antiviral drugs offer various advantages, including a shorter duration of sickness and a reduction in the intensity of symptoms. However, their effectiveness is most pronounced when administered early in the course of the illness. Additionally, the availability and accessibility of these drugs may vary by region, emphasizing the importance of consulting healthcare specialists.

Addressing Monkeypox Complications

Monkeypox, while often resolving on its own, may sometimes bring about complications that necessitate careful consideration. These complications can range in severity and may require medical intervention. Let's delve into a more detailed examination of potential issues and how to manage them.

Secondary Infections:

Monkeypox may lead to secondary bacterial infections on the skin. These infections, if left untreated, can escalate to more serious conditions. Swift and appropriate treatment with antibiotics is essential to address secondary infections promptly.

Eye Infections:

The virus can cause eye issues such as conjunctivitis or keratitis. In rare instances, these complications may result in visual impairment or even blindness. Seeking ophthalmic care as soon as any eye symptoms manifest is crucial to prevent and treat potential eye infections.

Respiratory Complications:

Severe cases of Monkeypox might give rise to respiratory discomfort or pneumonia. Timely medical intervention, including oxygen therapy and supportive care, is vital to uphold proper lung function and manage respiratory issues.

Swelling and Fluid Accumulation:

Certain Monkeypox patients may experience localized or systemic swelling, causing pain and, in severe cases, limiting movement. The treatment often involves the use of anti-inflammatory medications and compression garments to address edema effectively.

Scarring:

After the healing of Monkeypox lesions, scarring may occur, particularly in severe cases. While these scars generally fade over time, dermatological interventions, such as scar creams and laser therapy, can be employed to enhance their appearance.

Psychological Impact:

The emotional toll of Monkeypox should not be underestimated. The distress and worry associated with the disease may have lasting effects. Providing emotional support and therapy can prove valuable in helping patients and their families cope with psychological challenges.

It is essential to note that not every instance of Monkeypox will result in complications, and the severity can vary widely among individuals. Nonetheless, early detection and proactive measures are pivotal in managing complications effectively and mitigating their impact.

Preventing Complications:

The prevention of complications starts with providing robust supportive care and adhering to medical recommendations. This encompasses maintaining skin hygiene and avoiding scratching, thereby reducing the risk of subsequent infections. Adhering to the prescribed treatment plan is also crucial in preventing complications.

Ongoing Monitoring:

Individuals in the recovery phase from Monkeypox, particularly those with severe symptoms, should undergo regular monitoring to promptly identify and address any emerging problems. Healthcare professionals play a critical role in this continuous monitoring process.

Because of the restricted
human-to-human
transmission, effective
public health and
surveillance tactics can
assist contain outbreaks
and avoid widespread

Chapter 6: Outbreak Response and Public Health Measures

The goal of this chapter is to give you a detailed overview of the strategies and actions involved in managing this contagious illness.

Notifying and Watching

In any fight against infectious diseases, early detection and accurate reporting play a crucial role. This holds particularly true for Monkeypox. In this part, we'll delve into the details of reporting and monitoring during Monkeypox outbreaks.

Reporting Monkeypox Cases:

Promptly reporting Monkeypox cases is a key

part of the public health response. Both healthcare professionals and the general public have a responsibility to report. Whether you're a healthcare professional or a concerned citizen, if you suspect a Monkeypox case, it's crucial to inform the relevant authorities immediately. Quick notification can prevent further spread and enable a swift response.

Healthcare professionals play a vital role in this process, often being the first to encounter individuals with Monkeypox symptoms. Suspected cases should be reported to local health departments or national public health organizations. Medical expertise is essential to diagnose and confirm Monkeypox cases through laboratory testing.

The Significance of Surveillance:

Surveillance, like reporting, involves systematically collecting, analyzing, interpreting, and sharing health data. It helps authorities monitor the prevalence of the disease and identify trends in Monkeypox cases.

There are two types of surveillance: passive and active. Passive surveillance relies on healthcare personnel willingly reporting cases, a key method for tracking illnesses. Active surveillance, on the other hand, involves health professionals actively seeking potential cases, especially crucial in the early stages of an outbreak.

Tracing Contacts:

Contact tracing is closely linked to surveillance, as we'll see in the next section (6.2). It involves identifying and informing those who may have been exposed to the virus due to close contact with an affected person. These contacts are then monitored for symptoms and, if necessary, isolated to prevent the disease's spread.

Legal Framework: Legal frameworks exist at local, national, and international levels to support reporting and surveillance efforts. These laws establish the reporting and surveillance requirements and responsibilities of healthcare professionals, institutions, and the general public. Non-compliance with reporting obligations may have legal consequences due to the risk posed to public health.

It's essential to emphasize that these legal measures are not punitive but are in place to protect the public from the spread of contagious diseases like Monkeypox. These legal tools give public health authorities the ability to act in the best interests of public safety.

Contact Tracing

Imagine you find out you have Monkeypox. It's not only about your health but also about your family, friends, and anyone you've been around recently. Contact tracing is a reassuring and important plan in this situation.

Contact tracing is the careful process of finding, checking, and handling those who were close to someone with Monkeypox. It's not just for Monkeypox; it's a basic tool used to handle many infectious illnesses, like TB and certain infections.

What's Close Contact?

Close contact isn't just passing by someone on the street. It usually means spending a lot of time with or being close to an infected person. Close contact with Monkeypox could be living in the same house, taking care of an infected person, or having direct touch with their body fluids or sores.

How Contact Tracing Works: Contact tracing begins with the sick person. They are asked to list everyone they were around when they could spread the virus. This information is kept private and helps trace possible ways the virus could have spread.

Once found, these contacts are told about their possible exposure and the need for watching out for symptoms. This includes regular temperature checks and, if needed, staying away from others to avoid spreading the virus. The goal is to find new cases early and stop the spread.

Problems and Doing the Right Thing: Contact tracing has challenges and things to consider. Privacy and consent are very important. Those doing contact tracing must be careful with sensitive information and make sure people's rights and privacy are protected.

It's a balance between keeping people healthy and respecting their rights.

Also, contact tracing can take time. Trained people are needed to talk to contacts, give them information, and keep an eye on them. This can be tricky, especially in busy places. But the good part is that stopping the spread of sickness is more important than the challenges.

People in the Community: Getting the community involved is a big part of contact tracing. Building trust and working together is key to making this plan work. Communities need to understand why contact tracing is important for their health.

Controlling Monkeypox Globally

In our connected world, diseases like monkeypox don't stick to one place. When monkeypox outbreaks happen, local efforts might not be enough to reduce the risk. To stop the virus from spreading, improve healthcare systems, and help affected countries, everyone needs to work together on a global scale.

The Role of International Organizations: Groups like the World Health Organization (WHO) and the Centers for Disease Control and Prevention (CDC) are crucial in coordinating efforts worldwide to prevent monkeypox. They provide affected countries with technical knowledge, guidance, and resources. These organizations make sure we can track monkeypox cases globally by setting standard ways to diagnose and define cases.

They also help with monitoring, lab tests, and distributing medical supplies. Their involvement makes sure monkeypox is not just a local problem but a global one.

Research and Vaccine Development: Understanding the virus, how it spreads, and what causes it is crucial in global efforts to prevent monkeypox. International scientific cooperation helps with research on the virus and developing vaccines and treatments. Vaccination efforts in vulnerable areas and among at-risk groups can protect people from monkeypox, reducing the number of those who could get sick. Supporting research and vaccine development globally shows that we are committed to getting rid of the danger posed by this illness.

Training and Capacity Development: To make healthcare systems in affected areas better prepared, training and capacity development programs are essential. Providing healthcare staff with the right knowledge and skills ensures that monkeypox patients are taken care of effectively. These programs help local healthcare providers in diagnosing, treating, and preventing monkeypox. Building strong healthcare systems is an investment in public health, not just managing monkeypox.

International Response to Outbreaks: When monkeypox outbreaks happen, quick response teams from around the world can be sent to give emergency help. These teams can assist with tracking who came in contact with the virus, managing cases, and controlling infections. Their involvement strengthens local efforts and makes sure the outbreak is controlled as fast as possible.

Collaboration with Affected Countries: Global efforts against monkeypox rely on working together with countries that are affected. International organizations and partner governments join forces to support areas affected by providing financial and technical help. These partnerships aim to make places more resilient for future outbreaks and deal with the current crisis.

Conclusion

Thanks for checking out "Dealing with Monkey Pox: Prevention and Management."

We're glad you're interested in learning about Monkey Pox. This book aims to provide helpful info on understanding, preventing, and dealing with Monkey Pox outbreaks.

We hope the info here is helpful and interesting. Your commitment to staying informed contributes to the ongoing fight against infectious diseases.

If you enjoyed this book, consider exploring more from the author. Stay engaged, keep learning, and work towards a healthier, safer community.